Mental Health Holistic Approach

By
Paola Zanoni

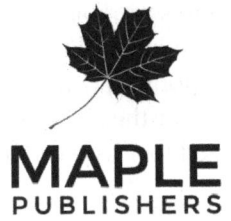

MAPLE
PUBLISHERS

Mental Health Holistic Approach

Author: Paola Zanoni

Copyright © 2024 Paola Zanoni

The right of Paola Zanoni to be identified as author of this work has been asserted by the author in accordance with section 77 and 78 of the Copyright, Designs and Patents Act 1988.

ISBN 978-1-83538-459-6 (Paperback)
   978-1-83538-460-2 (E-Book)

Book Cover Design and Layout by:
   White Magic Studios
   www.whitemagicstudios.co.uk

Published by:
   Maple Publishers
   Fairbourne Drive, Atterbury,
   Milton Keynes,
   MK10 9RG, UK
   www.maplepublishers.com

The views expressed in this work are solely those of the author and do not reflect the opinions of Publishers, and the Publisher hereby disclaims any responsibility for them. This book should not be used as a substitute for the advice of a competent authority, admitted or authorized to advise on the subjects covered.

Disclaimer

This booklet is supposed to be for information only.

I am not a doctor so please always seek professional advice.

My booklet aims to see mental illnesses under a more flexible and holistic approach against the rigidity of current medicine research and science, which influences mental illness issues and decisions in our society.

My wish is for you to find answers and inspiration on how to face these illnesses.

I hope you enjoy reading this booklet and my wish is for you to heal, manage, and improve your wellbeing.

Mental Health

There is a difference between being born with a mental illness and becoming mentally ill.

The difference is that if you become mentally ill you can heal and fully recover, however if you are born with it, depending on the pathology and nature of the person, people can improve using techniques which will help them to cope better with themselves and the outside world.

First, let's define mental illnesses typologies and explain what they really are.

Narcissism

I am going to describe narcissism under a Human point of view. By this I mean how Humans perceive narcissism behaviour.

Narcissism is not a mental illness, it is a race and you are born narcissist, you don't become narcissist. Keeping in mind that narcissists, no matter who they are or which country they are from in the world, they have the same patterns in behaviour.

Under a Mental Health point of view based on science Narcissistic Personality Disorder (NPD) is considered a mental health condition that includes an unhealthy sense of self-importance and a need for admiration. People with NPD lack empathy and have difficulty forming genuine emotional connections.

According to Mental Health studies, the main negative traits of narcissistic behaviour are:

They have a strong sense of entitlement, often they expect special treatment and privileges.

They lack empathy and they are unable to recognize the needs and feelings of others.

Often they will act as in taking advantage of others to get what they want.

They can become envious of others, especially when others are successful, They focus a lot on wealth, power, beauty, or brilliance.

They tend a lot to view themselves as they are special or unique although often they lack self-esteem, doubting themselves or feeling empty.

They are very sensitive to criticism, often reacting badly to disagreements or confrontations.

According to science there are few psychotherapy techniques that can help people with NPD to learn to manage their symptoms.

These are Talk Therapy, which helps people learn to relate to others, understand their feelings, and recognize their strengths and weaknesses. Another two common therapies are Dialectical Behavioral Therapy (DBT) and Cognitive Behavioral Therapy (CBT) which are common type of therapies for NPD which are therapies that help to deal with overwhelming problems in a more positive way in order to break down problems into smaller parts; these include thoughts, feelings and actions of the patient. By this the patient learns techniques to change unhelpful thoughts and behaviours into more healthy ones. Other useful therapies according to science are Transference-Focused Psychotherapy (TFP) which is a more structured type of therapy that helps people work on feelings in a safe environment; and last there is Gestalt Therapy which is a type of therapy that focuses on the present and how past experiences can affect people's feelings.

Under an holistic point of view however narcissists can be good people. It depends a lot on the level of self-awareness they have and the effort they want to put into trying to understand and manage their own needs and behaviors. Many can be generous, kind, and loyal to those they care about. They can also be successful, driven, and ambitious.

In my opinion there are different levels of narcissism behaviour; however narcissists are becoming more empathic, some can be very caring and loving and this is also because narcissistic people have a clear inner understanding of what is right and wrong.

The bible tells how Jewish people were bad to each other while crossing the desert. This is the reason Moses instituted the 10 commandments to create a code of conduct for the Jewish, and this is when the first laws were created to protect people. Narcissists follow the rules as they have a good understanding of right and wrong. With the 10 commandments we also have the first development of bureaucracy.

In conclusion, narcissism is a race. They show up in every country under every nationality and religion. They can be very fascinating and interesting. They have very good points and they are very persuasive and captivating. We live in a world governed by narcissistics laws (which are needed). However these laws can be used by people in power against normal humans and even against narcissists themselves, and toward all the people who behave out of good intentions - also this current society unfortunately promotes the very unhealthy narcissistic behaviour, which is one of the causes of corruption in our society.

My suggestion is always to encourage empathy and behave out of empathy and good intentions. Narcissists are very curious about love, they know it is good. They will encourage it and promote love. Narcissists don't feel emotions, they feel through you, through common humans; however their strong point is that they have very clear understanding of what is right and wrong which can help them a lot to become good people and improve the quality standards of life and health too.

Narcissists can show lots of confidence and charm which can be appealing to people to draw attention towards them. They are ambitious and they can have a strong drive for success and achievement.

However as I have explained previously these people are very charismatic and fascinating. Thanks to their nature, narcissist are very skilled technically and they have introduced many good things in the world. These people, contrary to Human nature who are people who have more creative tendencies, are very technical and have contributed to society with lots of new and positive innovations and also brought order within people with the creation of rules and laws which are very important to established order in society.

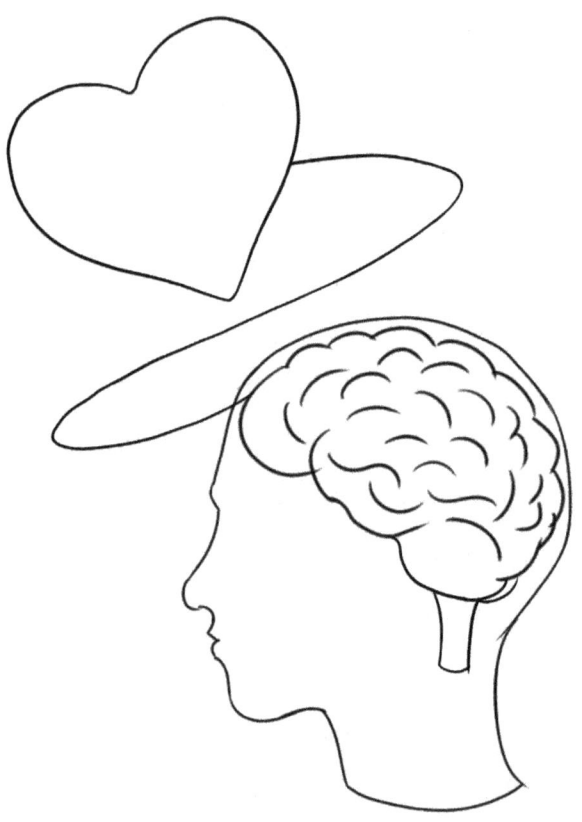

Psychopath – Antisocial Personality Disorder

Psychopath disorder apparently affects more females. Doctors officially diagnose people with the term antisocial personality disorder. You are born with this mental disorder and it is genetic. Often close family members suffer from the disorder themselves. This may aggravate the mental state of their kids. For example, carers may misuse alcohol or drugs and neglect or abuse their kids or have inconsistent parenting approaches toward their children.

This disorder is one of the most challenging types of personality disorder. These people's behaviour can be impulsive, irresponsible and often dishonest and also they might engage in criminal behaviour.

Usually these people are manipulative, deceitful, and reckless, and will not care for other people's feelings. They don't care about rules, the law or the rights of others. They may tell lies, behave aggressively or violently, and also steal. Psychopaths are goal oriented; they are unwilling to control impulses or delay gratification. These people often use rage to control people and to manipulate them into submission. They lack empathy, often they are sadistic as in taking pleasure in inflicting pain on their victims or in deceiving them to the point that they even find it funny. They lack concern, regret and remorse about other people's distress. They lack guilt and they don't learn from their mistakes. On top of it, they blame others for the problems in their lives. Psychopaths are not able to form healthy relationships; they disregard society and its conventions, values and norms.

Psychopaths are keen to make secret plans to deceive others, are calculative, ruthless and long term career criminals and often their behaviour is premeditated and cunning.

These people often can suffer from anxiety and depression symptoms. There are different forms of therapy that are used to monitor antisocial personality disorder although it is never totally cured. The first one is Cognitive Behaviour Therapy which is a talking therapy that helps to manage the way these people think and behave. Another interesting therapy in use is Mentalisation Based Therapy. This is another talking therapy and it has become popular in dealing with psychopath disorder as it helps to understand thoughts, beliefs, wishes and feelings and to link these to actions and therefore improve behaviour. The goal of this therapy is for these people to understand what's going on in their minds and in the minds of other people as consequence to their behaviour and to link these understandings to improve problematic behaviour. The point of this therapy is to focus how these people think and try to understand how their mental state affects their behaviour. Another therapy approach often used is Democratic Therapeutic Communities and this is based on a group of people with the same pathology in engaging in activities and while they get help they help others too. So, for example, this might be people living in a community home where they all have rules: one cooking, one doing the garden, one tidying etc. Under these premises these people can change, unfold and be more aware of their own behaviour.

Apparently there is little evidence that medication can help these people; however antipsychotic and antidepressant might be recommended sometimes.

Often these people can have mental health disorders such as depression and anxiety and they engage in substance and alcohol misuse that can aggravate behaviour.

There is some evidence that these people's behaviour is similar to the so-called in Narcissism language the **"flying monkeys"**. There is also evidence that these flying monkeys have lots of characteristics similar to those of the Spider monkeys - Spider monkeys belong to the Atelidae family which are one of the families recognised as the New World monkeys (new world as in Central and South America new continents). These monkeys are larger than average and this family of monkeys include four types of female monkeys, as detailed below. Additionally, there are four male variants, each with a typology distinct from that of the females.

Howler monkey, they have earned their name from the loud noise they produce with their throat, another characteristic of these monkeys is their wide, round nostrils.

<u>Spider monkey</u>, they are called like this because they have long arms long as their legs and their skin underneath the thick hair is black,

<u>Woolly monkeys</u> are called like this because they have short woolly hair, long limbs and a long prehensile tail.

<u>Woolly spider monkey</u>, also known as muriquis. This last one is the larger of the family - it's huge compare to the others. This is why murquis in native Tupi means "largest monkey" and the characteristics of this monkey is that they are more leisure orientated as they spend an average of 49% of their day resting.

The "flying monkeys" is a term in psychology that comes from the Wizard of Oz, a book by L. Frank Baum. In the story these monkeys have been enslaved by the Wicked Witch - originally they were called the Winged monkey.

From a mental illness point of view flying monkeys refers to a person such as an abuser or a psychopath who are submissive themselves to a psychopath or even a narcissist or a energy vampire. Their task is usually to help energy vampires to extend control over friends, family members or other narcissists by, for example, harassing victims, twisting the truth, being dishonest, playing the victim, sending threats and also using violence.

Sociopath – Antisocial Personality Disorder

Sociopaths apparently are more males and they have the same diagnosis as psychopaths which is antisocial personality disorder; however there are a few differences between the two.

The main difference between sociopaths and psychopaths is that sociopaths have an understanding of what is right and wrong while psychopaths don't have the ability to distinguish right from wrong; apparently sociopaths have a conscience, which is a moral sense of right and wrong, and often try to justify themselves for some wrongdoing as they are aware they are doing wrong to someone; while psychopaths believe their actions are justified and they feel no remorse or guilt for action when they are harming others.

Sociopaths tend to act more impulsively than psychopaths; however they struggle to accomplish long term goals such as keep a job where psychopaths are more able to accomplish long term goals. When it comes to relationships sociopaths may be able to keep long term relationships with like-minded people while psychopaths struggle to form long term attachments. Other differences are while sociopaths make it clear they don't care for others and their behaviour can be hot-headed and impulsive psychopaths pretend to care and their behaviour is cold-hearted. Sociopaths rationalise and recognise what they are doing while psychopaths maintain a normal life as a cover for their criminal activities.

It seems the medical approach and techniques to manage sociopaths disorder is the same as for psychopaths disorder listed above; however this is done taking into consideration the differences between the two personality disorders.

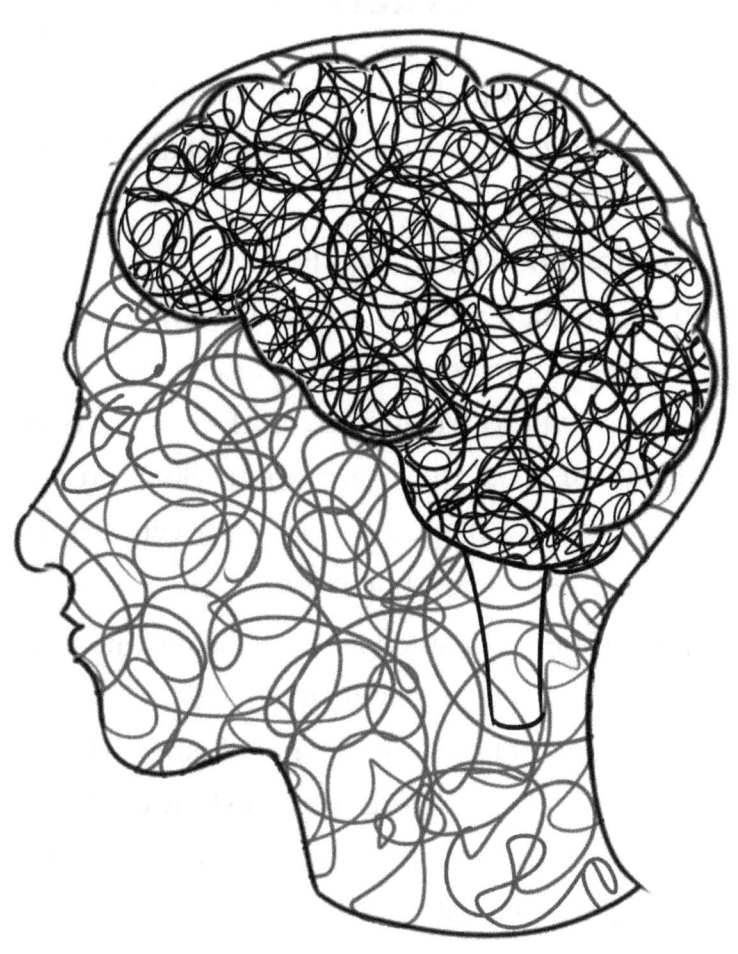

Borderline

Borderlines are all female - I think there exists a kind of the male version but it's a totally different topic.

You don't become borderline, you are born like that -these women are very messed up in their head and I am going to explain this below - apparently there are 5 types/variation of borderlines. To my knowledge in total there are about 3050 women borderline on the planet; this is not a very reliable figure though - but could be close.

Borderline is classified as a personality disorder. These women who are affected have many toxic behaviour traits. These traits are mainly shown in how they relate to others. These women show emotional instability called also affective dysregulation. They show also disturbed patterns of thinking or perception - often they engage in impulsive behaviour and also they tend to have intense but unstable types of relationships especially with males.

These women often experience intensive negative emotions such as rage, sorrow, shame, panic, terror, long-term feelings of emptiness and loneliness, including mood swings and often feel even suicidal.

They have thoughts - they are a terrible person and try to find reassurance around them that these thoughts are not truth - sometimes these women engage in irresponsible activities such as drinking, drug misuse, spending or gambling, impulsive sex with strangers.

Often they feel unsure between abandonment and getting too close so they would be constantly texting and phoning a partner - or calling them in the middle of the night - clinging and refusing to let go a person - threatening to harm or kill themselves if the person leaves them.

Often they have these love-hate relationships with their partners - these women often seem to have a very rigid "black & white" view of relationships and they would emotionally confuse their partners with mixed signals as "go away/please don't go" states of mind - behaviour that often can lead to break-ups.

Borderline is not cured with medication but instead with individual and group psychotherapy. These types of therapies can help to resolve problems and to change their attitudes and behaviour toward those problems; as a good therapist would explain, the right approach to face certain issues is for these women to learn to establish what is considered right and what is considered wrong especially from an emotional point of view. I believe this approach would help to validate their emotions (as often partners don't know how to deal with these women mainly out of confusion) especially to find reassurances as these women tend to feel often very fragile and insecure about their feelings and how they are perceived by others.

These women are constantly dealing with a mix of contrasting emotions which makes them very insecure and fragile and a good talking therapy with a therapist or even a group therapy could help them to put an order between feeling and reality - as how you should feel in a particular situation according to common sense.

There is DBT as in Dialectical Behaviour Therapy specifically designed to treat people with Borderline symptoms.

The goal of this therapy is to validate emotions and to teach the women to be more flexible and not to see everything under the black and white glasses but instead with grey shades too. The idea is to help them free from destructive behaviour as these women tend to see the world, relationships and life in a very rigid way, according to research. I would add - probably this is specific on making decisions. Their frame of mind in making decisions would sound like "shall we go to the cinema or move to another country?" However, when it comes to dealing with people they go "over the border-line" in the sense that they don't respect boundaries or ethic rules.

There are other types of psychotherapy techniques as:

Mentalisation-based therapy where mentalisation is the ability to think and examine your own thoughts and beliefs and assess whether they are useful and realistic. Another therapy is Therapeutic communities (TCs), these are structured group environments where people are taught skills to interact socially with others - also Art therapies are useful to help people to express their emotions through art.

As I have mentioned earlier, one of these women's main characteristics is that they are abusive to men and tend to treat them badly - especially mentally and emotionally. Some borderline females who are very cruel push men to an extent to make them become sick or even feel suicidal. Many of these women are very captivating and charming and very beautiful however they are very messed up especially regarding boundaries - right and wrong - respect - approach to other women and approach to men, especially in relationships.

Under the holistic point of view, borderline women are said to have gifts due to their nature as telekinesis or telepathy, spell casting, cursing even divine healing powers as in disease reduction and healing aura.

Often, under an holistic point of view, these women are defined as the sirens from the book of Homer, The Odyssey. Here Odysseus encounters the sirens at one point on his travels. The story tells of how he defeats the siren's allurings. He tells his crew to put wax in their ears and to tie him to the mast so he was the only one who could hear them. He also tells his crew to ignore wherever he is saying and to not untie him. Sirens often are portrayed as bad in mythology because they were leading sailors to their death.

This phenomenon currently happens with men who have been in relationships with these types of women. Even after relationships are ended, (we are talking under an holistic approach to this mental illness here) they use their telepathy and telekinesis abilities to torment their exes sometimes to the point of pushing them to suicidal. Men are affected mentally by these women. Sometimes they describe seeing images of these women's faces in their minds, some men describe their feeling as "they feel they are drowning".

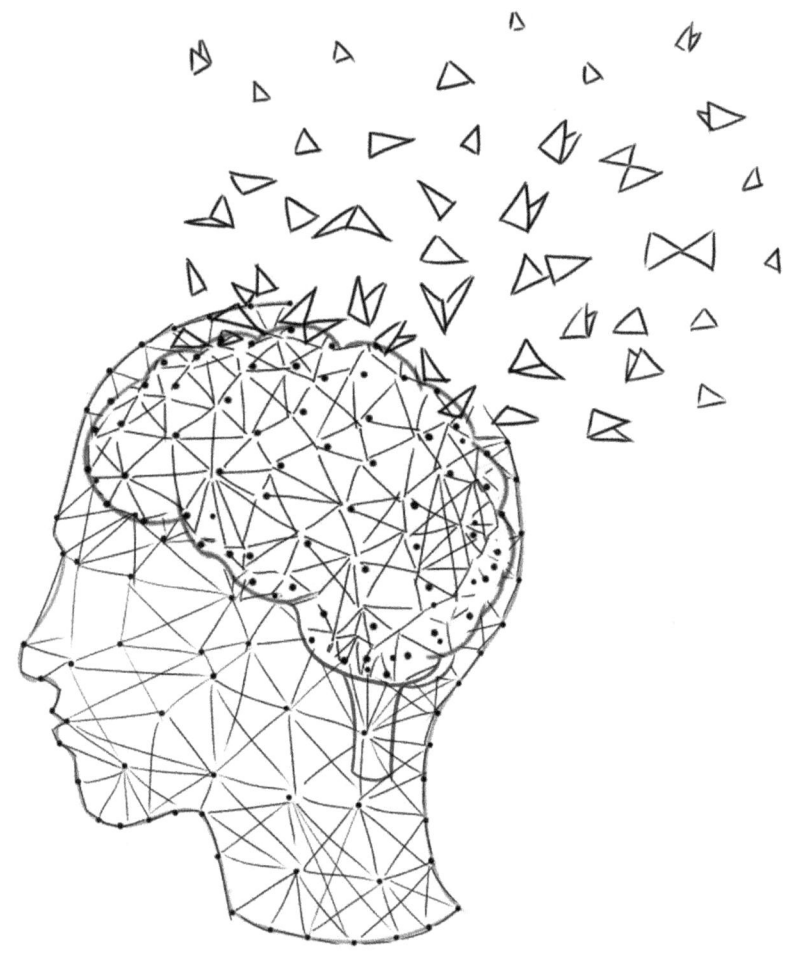

Bipolarism

This is a topic I know very little about - as there is a lot of info but it can get quite tricky and confusing.

The main characteristic of bipolar disorder is the rapid change in moods from strong highs to strong lows. Bipolar would experience periods of extreme high energy and activity, these symptoms are called manic episodes and symptoms could include confusion, disorientation, losing the need of sleep and irritability. These symptoms are alternated with periods of extreme sadness and are called depressive episodes some of the symptoms are a loss of interest in activities once enjoyed, feeling very tired, difficulty in concentrating or remembering things, and in some extreme cases even thinking or considering suicide.

The causes of bipolar disorder are unclear. However my theory is that we could be dealing with people with high sensitiveness to the environment as their mood swings can be affected by season changes and there is some literature that claims by moon phases - although research is still needed on this, season changes but also moon phases seem to affect bipolarism.

Apparently light therapy can help with symptoms - during light therapy you are exposed to artificial lights. As in supplements Omega 3 can help a lot with bipolarism although you need to take it at least for six months before seeing results. Omega 3 helps especially with low moods; also helps a lot in the reduction of symptoms such as irritability and anxiety as it helps increase serotonin release and also helps improving mood relaxation.

There are some theories that explain that bipolarism might be linked to genetics as it seems it run in families. It also seems stressful situations such as breakdown of a relationship, abuse or a death of a loved one might trigger symptoms. Problems in everyday life such as money, work, relationships, sleep disturbances patterns and also physical illnesses trigger people with bipolar disorder.

Bipolarism is mainly treated with medication such as mood stabilisers like lithium, a combination -of antipsychotics and antidepressants -??, and anti-anxiety medication. Often medication is in combination with psychotherapy such as talking therapies. Also keeping a balanced lifestyle such as regular exercise, planning enjoyable daily or weekly activities, good diet and healthy sleep patterns can help to live a more healthier life.

What I know about bipolarism is that they are extremely intelligent and capable of grandiose things, but then there is the other side of the coin where at times they feel very powerless and low in moods.

Hashimoto's disease

There is evidence in science researches that often Hashimoto's disease has been misdiagnosed with bipolar disorder and it seems this happens often; in fact just in 1987, 15% of patients admitted to psychiatric hospital were misdiagnosed with mental illnesses where actually they were suffering from hypothyroidism (Hashimoto's thyroiditis). *(Is it mental illness or Hashimoto's Thyroiditis? 2020).*

Hashimoto's thyroiditis, also known as chronic lymphocytic thyroiditis or Hishimotos' disease, is an autoimmune disease in which the thyroid gland is slowly destroyed. Over time some people might develop symptoms and weight gain, depression, and general pain. Hashimoto's thyroiditis further complications can be high cholesterol, heart disease, heart failure and high blood pressure etc.

Some of the symptoms of Hashimoto's disease related to mental health are anxiety, panic attacks, insomnia, difficulty concentrating or thinking clearly, confusion and forgetfulness; weakness and fatigue, feeling excessively cold or hot, depression and an overall swing in symptoms and therefore in moods.

Mental Health Holistic Approach

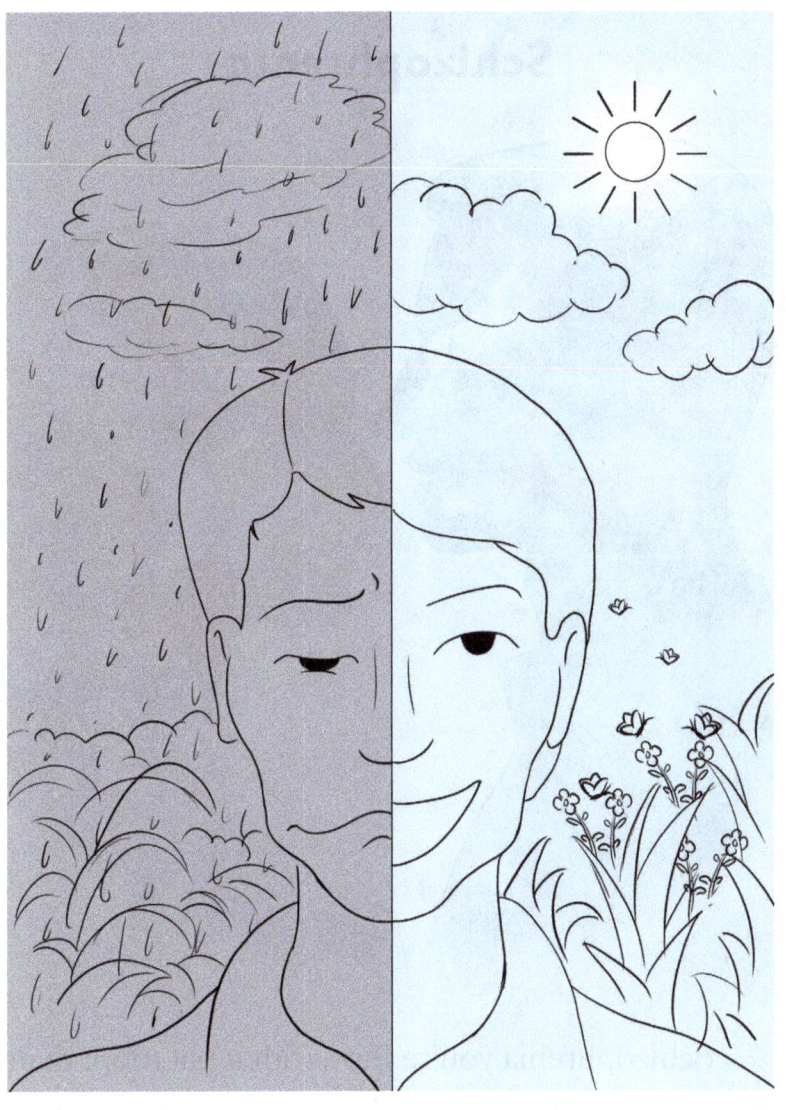

Schizophrenia

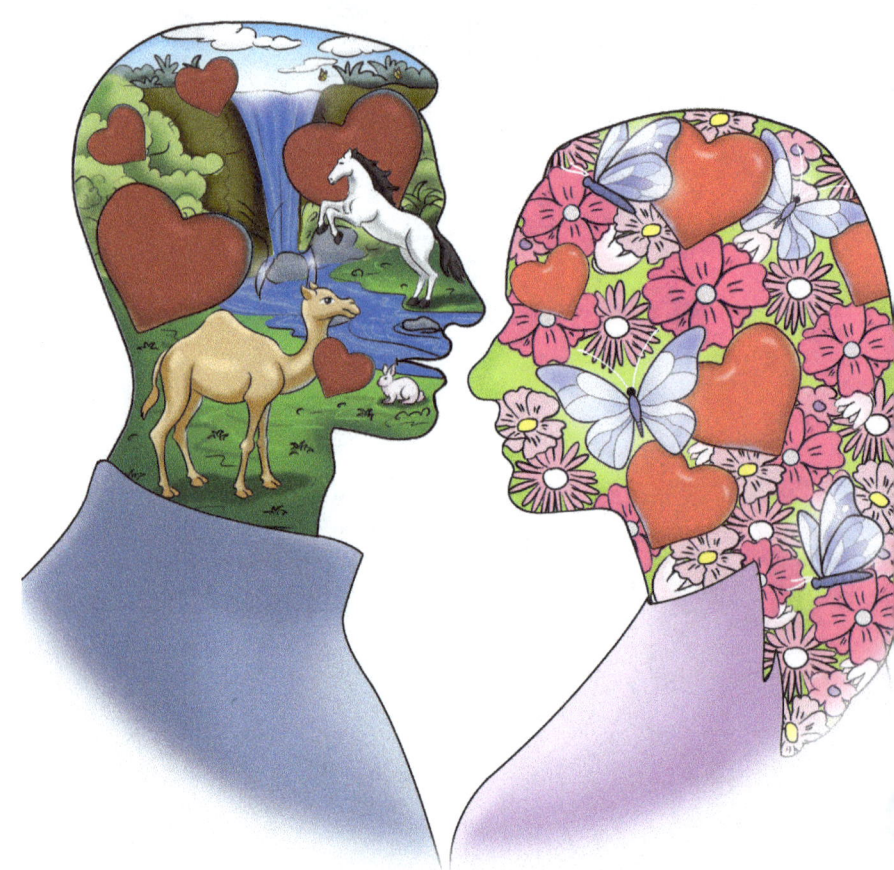

Schizophrenia you're born with it but more than being classified as a mental illness I would say is an intellect power or gift if you learn how to manage it. This especially when you have the first symptoms and break through which can be unexpected and traumatic. If you don't know how to channel them you can end up easily in psychosis and medication might be required to numb the sudden confusion and sometimes even hospitalisation is needed. Often with schizophrenia you can have psychotic symptoms which means sometimes a person may end up in a state of confusion as they might not be able to distinguish their own inner thoughts from the voices in their heads. This might affect decisions making which can come across as random; if these symptoms are not channelled and acknowledged the person can find themselves in a state of total confusion.

Science says most people with schizophrenia make a recovery although few might experience some occasional return of psychosis. Current treatments to manage symptoms are talking therapies, cognitive behaviour therapy, arts therapy, medication usually antipsychotic medication. In my understanding antipsychotic medicines are actually anaesthetic, similar to the ones used in operations, when you are put to sleep. This medication numbs your feelings and slower your thoughts and therefore your symptoms. It is important to manage symptoms and maintain a healthy lifestyle including exercise, good sleeping patterns and healthy diet.

However under a holistic point of view some of the voices that schizophrenic people claim to hear, can actually be telepathy as in becoming one with the universal consciousness due to the opening of the third chakra. Often this is associated with intuition, perception and deeper consciousness - the emotion associated with this phenomenon is compassion. It seems also other phenomena associated with these feelings are spirituality, wisdom, devotion, creativity, justice, impartiality and dignity. As mentioned earlier, it seems people subject to these awakening symptoms are subject to the opening of the brow chakra (third eye) which controls the pineal gland. The pineal gland (pineal meaning literally shaped like a pine cone) is also called "third eye" and is located in the centre of the brain. The pineal gland releases the highest level of melatonin when there is darkness and lower level of melatonin when you are exposed to light. Melatonin plays an important role in the body with sleeping patterns, feeling relaxed and calm.

From an holistic point of view, activating the pineal gland can lead to a high intuition, clarity of thoughts, and an increased awareness of one's surroundings. When the third eye is opened, intuition increases, there is a higher sensitivity to energy, enhanced perception, vivid dreams, and it improves the sense of synchronicity in your life.

This phenomenon can happen suddenly. The symptoms can be quite frightening if you are not aware of this holistic approach and the person affected might enter a state of confusion and panic, this is also called in science - psychosis.

As a solution it would be useful to learn to channel and control the symptoms. People should do this by taking time to listen to their inner voices and focus on their mind and body, internal and external symptoms. Mainly Humans are affected by this pathology.

Spectrum Autism – Adhd – Asperger's And The Indigo Kids

You are born with it. There are a lot of theories about the "Indigo Children" around as a new phenomenon, as seeing these kids actually not through the eyes of a disability but actually as if they have some intellect powers and gifts. Some people claim these kids are an evolution of the human race and messengers of the world.

These children often have socialisation problems. They are hyperactive, very sensitive, rebel against any form of authority. They have great inner strength, are highly creative, highly empathic, they have strong intellectual faculties such as memory, reason, intuition, perception and imagination. They have a high sense of morality which means good principles concerning the distinction between right and wrong or good and bad. Strong morality examples are - being honest, treating others with respect, helping others, and strong technology skills.

One curiosity is that Indigo is a colour of the spectrum. Under a holistic point of view Indigo's meaning is great devotion, wisdom and justice including fairness and impartiality. Often indigo is associated with intuition, perception and deeper consciousness - the emotion associated with indigo is compassion. It seems also indigo is a calming colour of the spectrum which symbolises spirituality, wisdom, devotion, creativity, justice, impartiality and dignity. Indigo links with the brow chakra (third eye) and controls the pineal gland. The pineal gland (pineal meaning literally shaped like a pine cone) is also called "third eye" and is located in the centre of the brain - the pineal gland releases the highest level of melatonin when there is darkness and lower level of melatonin when you are exposed to light- melatonin plays an important role in the body with sleeping patterns, feeling relaxed and calm. From a holistic point of view, activating the pineal gland can lead to a high intuition, clarity of thoughts, and an increased awareness of one's surroundings. When the third eye is open, intuition increases, there is a higher sensitivity to energy, enhanced perception, vivid dreams, and it improves the sense of synchronicity in your life.

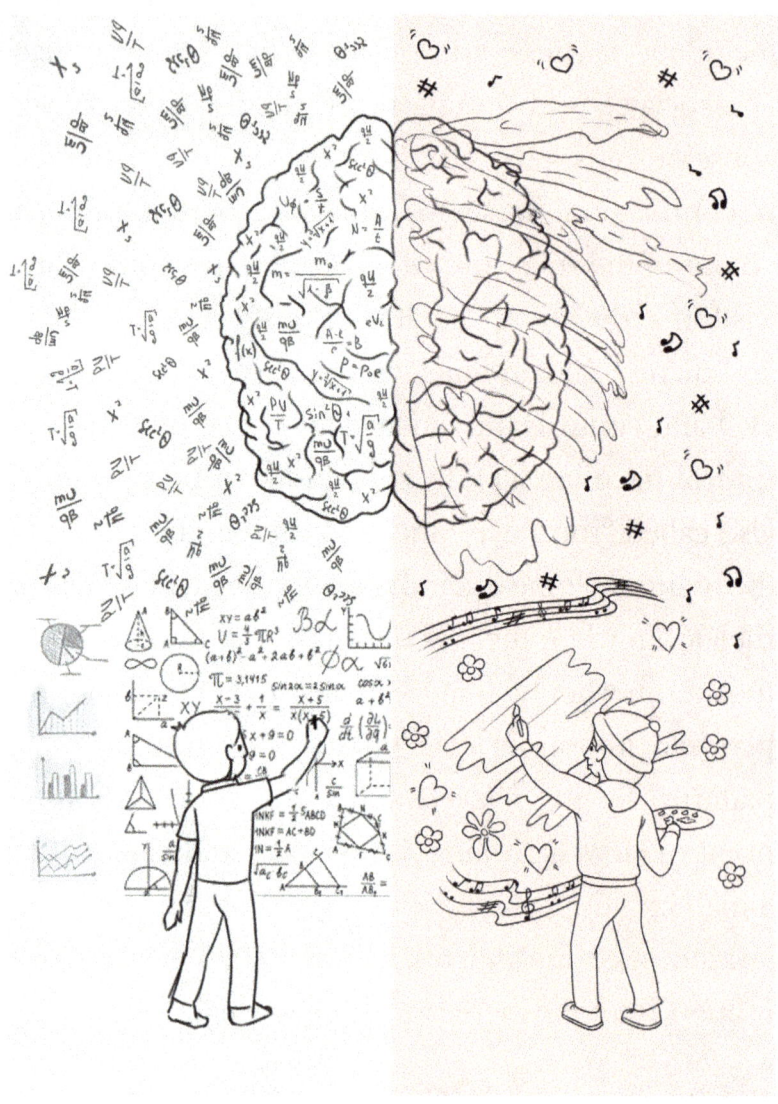

Ptsd – Post Traumatic Stress Disorder

PTSD is the cause of a distressing, frightening, or a traumatic event experienced during the course of someone's life. These could be serious accidents, physical or sexual assault, domestic violence, child abuse, a serious health problem, sudden death of someone close, war and conflict as for example combat veterans.

Often symptoms develop during the first few months of the traumatic episode but there have been cases where they showed delays of months or even years before first symptoms are shown. Some of these symptoms are flashbacks, nightmares, distressing images and physical sensations such as feeling sick, heart rate accelerating, sweating etc. Often these people feel anxious and easily irritable, they have sleeping problems and they find it hard to concentrate. They also experience symptoms such as headaches, dizziness, chest and stomach aches. Often they develop other problems such as depression, anxiety and phobias.

PTSD can in few cases cause paranoia; often the person can become irrationally suspicious of others. They can become very hypervigilant, this is also called fight-or-flight state where they live in a constant state of panic and suspiciousness of people and their motives. Especially when they are in a relationship are always expecting a betrayal and they are constantly looking for clues and reading between the lines when talking to people. The paranoia symptoms together with PTSD are associated to people who have had a long term relationship with an abusive partner, for example a narcissist (partners, family member and so on) who often have gaslighted the victim; therefore their reaction of hypervigilance and panic-like symptoms which they might show as increase in heart rate, sweat and increase of body temperature. These symptoms are manifested, especially when they feel exposed or close to the trauma trigger.

People with PTSD often deal with it by avoiding talking about the trauma experience, pushing memories away or avoiding talking about the episode.

Some people isolate themselves and withdraw from activities they used to enjoy. Some people would describe their emotions as feeling numb. Many deal with symptoms by self-harm or toxic destructive behaviour engaging in drugs and alcohol misuse.

C-PTSD - complex post-traumatic stress disorder - In this case the trauma is a long-term traumatic experience where the person finds it difficult or impossible to escape or avoid. These includes child abuse or neglect, domestic violence, living in war zone, being a prisoner of war, witnessing violence and abuse for a long time or being forced into prostitution etc. The person, on top of the symptoms of PTSD, also has extreme problems with managing emotions and relationships and in general they have problems in dealing with people in a healthy way.

Most popular treatments of PTSD and CPTSD are talking therapy. An example is Cognitive Behavioural Therapy (CBT); with this approach therapists use techniques to cope and come to terms with the traumatic episode. The point is to help to process the trauma memories so over time symptoms will fade away.

EMDR (Eye Movement Desensitisation and Reprocessing) is another apparently very effective technique to deal with PTSD and CPTSD. It consists of talking through the traumatic episode in detail while the therapist encourages the patient to make eye movement by following the fingers of the therapist. This therapy also includes tapping on the patient's hands or front thighs- (there is also a self-help technique called butterfly where the patient with arms crossed taps himself on the chest on alternative beats). The way this therapy works is that apparently the trauma is stored in the right part of the brain in the amygdala. The therapist, by the finger movement in front of the eyes of the client and also the tapping, helps the trauma to be released and to expand to the left part too. It seems with the help of the tapping, but also eye movement and by the patient discussing the incident at the same time, slowly the trauma releases its strength and becomes a memory. In this case, the strong emotions of the trauma are normalized and they do not affect the patient anymore. This can be done in just a few sessions depending on the trauma or traumas of the client. With this technique, the trauma is not emotionally painful anymore and it becomes just a bad memory and it doesn't trigger the person anymore.

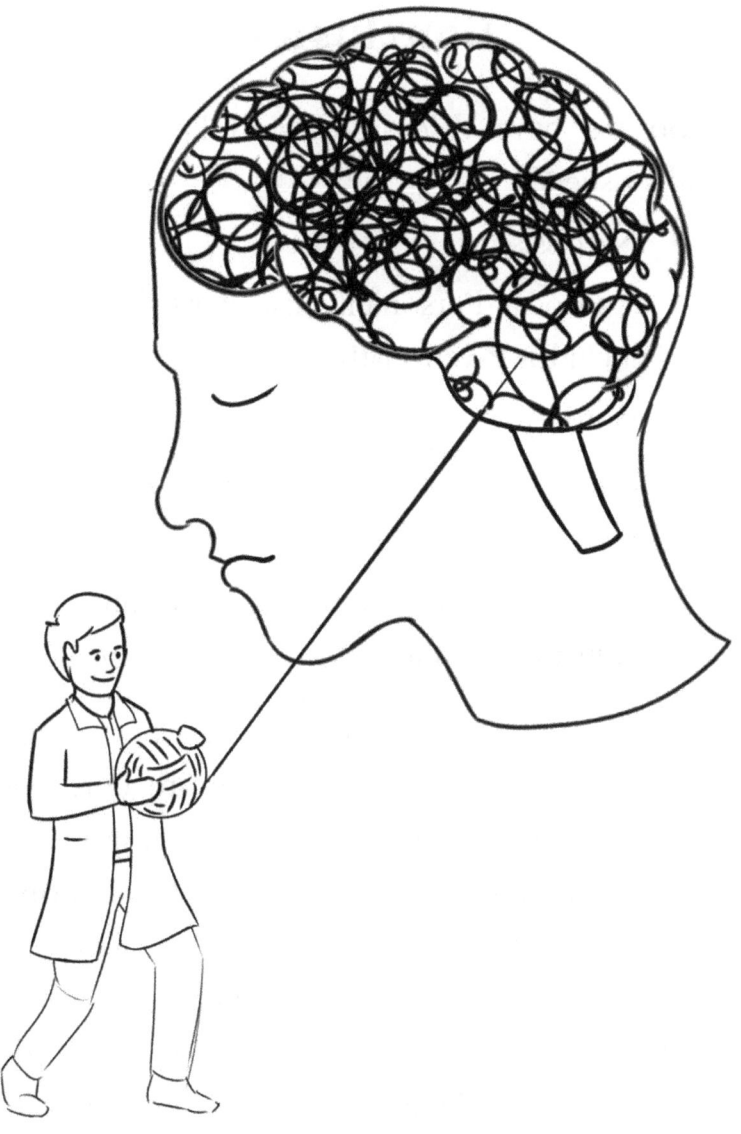

Conclusion

So we have discussed the following mental healths issue:

- Narcissism
- Antisocial Personality disorder (which includes Psychopath and Sociopath)
- Borderline
- Bipolarism (including Hashimoto's disease)
- Schizofrenia
- Indigo Kids (which include Spectrum Autism, Adhd and Asperger's Syndrome)

Regarding the mental illnesses above, according to my understanding, some people are born with them, others might have a predisposition which can develop during the course of their lives. As I described in the introduction there are certain mental illnesses which you are born with and others you become ill during the course of your life. As I have explained if you become mentally ill you can fully recover but if you are born with it (and this includes not only the off-side symptoms but also the perks that comes with each illness) depending on the pathology and nature of the person, people can improve using techniques which will help them to manage every day lives better. At the end of the day we all want to feel good within ourselves and the outside world.

Then we have got PTSD (Post Traumatic Stress Disorder) and CPTSD (Complex Post Traumatic Stress Disorder)

You are not born with this - this mental illness is a consequence of major or minor traumas people have experienced during the course of their lives. You can recuperate from PTSD and CPTSD with proper therapy, a healthy lifestyle and inner work. According to the gravity of the trauma sometimes therapy can take longer than others. I believe everybody on this planet on some extent is affected by PTSD.

Then we have symptoms which in a bizarre way we all experience despite the nature of the illness. These, however, are experienced on a different scale according to the person affected. Some of these symptoms are anxiety, stress, panic attacks, social anxiety, compulsive disorders and depression.

Under an holistic point of view I would like to define the above mentioned mental illness (excluding PTSD and CPTSD) as races and I will explain why below.

People are born with certain characteristics and I believe it is due to their DNA and genes why they are affected by one instead of another - So I would define these mental illnesses as races. The reason why they are one type or another is according to their ancestors and their family DNA.

Under an holistic point of view there are other two mental illness or races as I like to call them, that I haven't mentioned in this booklet and these are the Energy Vampires and the Reptilians, (these mental illness are here mentioned by the races under an holistic point of view) which I might discuss in a future book.

In conclusion this booklet doesn't only have to be viewed as a mental-holistic to understand diagnosis but also as a sociology book with the intention also to help people to understand society and its habitants.

Bibliography

- https://en.wikipedia.org/wiki/Narcissism
- https://www.nhs.uk/mental-health/conditions/borderline-personality-disorder/overview/
- https://superpowerfanon.fandom.com/wiki/Nymph_Physiology
- https://www.healthline.com/health/bipolar-disorder/bipolar-mood-episode-triggers#life-events
- https://www.nhs.uk/mental-health/conditions/bipolar-disorder/overview/
- https://psychcentral.com/bipolar/full-moon-bipolar-disorder#tips
- https://holtorfmed.com/articles/is-it-mental-illness-or-hashimotos-thyroiditis/#:~:text=This%20can%20cause%20depression%2C%20weight,it%20happens%20much%20too%20often.

- https://en.wikipedia.org/wiki/Hashimoto%27s_thyroiditis
- https://www.nhs.uk/mental-health/conditions/borderline-personality-disorder/overview/
- https://powerlisting.fandom.com/wiki/Nymph_Physiology
- https://www.nhsinform.scot/illnesses-and-conditions/mental-health/schizophrenia/
- https://www.studiocataldi.it/articoli/41210-il-linguaggio-dell-autismo.asp
- https://www.nostrofiglio.it/bambino/psicologia/bambini-indaco
- https://www.amazon.co.uk/Indigo-Children-Kids-Have-Arrived/dp/1561706086
- https://www.nhs.uk/mental-health/conditions/antisocial-personality-disorder/
- https://alouattasen.weebly.com/uploads/8/9/5/6/8956452/spidermonkeycare.pdf
- https://en.m.wikipedia.org/wiki/Atelidae
- https://www.verywellmind.com/what-is-a-sociopath-380184

- https://www.phoenix-society.org/resources/calming-trauma
- https://www.nhs.uk/mental-health/conditions/post-traumatic-stress-disorder-ptsd/overview/
- https://www.nimh.nih.gov/health/publications/post-traumatic-stress-disorder-ptsd

www.ingramcontent.com/pod-product-compliance
Lightning Source LLC
Chambersburg PA
CBHW070036040426
42333CB00040B/1699